ANXIETY

How to Overcome Couple Conflicts and Jealousy

(Overcome Stressful Anxiety With These Emotional Healing Tools)

Walter Smith

Published by Oliver Leish

Walter Smith

All Rights Reserved

*Anxiety: How to Overcome Couple Conflicts and Jealousy
(Overcome Stressful Anxiety With These Emotional Healing
Tools)*

ISBN 978-1-77485-233-0

Legal & Disclaimer

The information contained in this book is not designed to replace or take the place of any form of medicine or professional medical advice. The information in this book has been provided for educational and entertainment purposes only.

The information contained in this book has been compiled from sources deemed reliable, and it is accurate to the best of the Author's knowledge; however, the Author cannot guarantee its accuracy and validity and cannot be held liable for any errors or omissions. Changes are periodically made to this book. You must consult your doctor or get professional medical advice before using any of the suggested remedies, techniques, or information in this book.

Upon using the information contained in this book, you agree to hold harmless the Author from and against any damages, costs, and expenses, including any legal fees potentially resulting from the application of any of the information provided by this guide. This disclaimer applies to any damages or injury caused by the use and application, whether directly or indirectly, of any advice or information presented, whether for breach of contract, tort, negligence, personal injury, criminal intent, or under any other cause of action.

You agree to accept all risks of using the information presented inside this book. You need to consult a professional medical practitioner in order to ensure you are both able and healthy enough to participate in this program.

TABLE OF CONTENTS

Introduction

The world is extremely chaotic. There's too much happening and it's easy to get lost in the chaos. The issue is that the majority of people are so focused on their past and future that they don't think about the present, allowing their lives to slip by.

What Is Mindfulness?

Mindfulness is the state of being in which a person is able to be completely aware of what does regardless of what's happening. This skill can be observed in certain individuals, however it is something that is attainable by anyone who wants to have more control over their lives.

Have you heard of an autopilot?

If a machine is operating in autopilot mode, it allows less control by the human operator. Unfortunately, there are people who are operating on autopilot. They spend their time doing nothing but routines in the name of an insanity. It's a common practice however this doesn't mean that it's appropriate for everyone. When you're not fully in the moment it's like you've lost the feeling of living. It's as if you're not living life in the first place.

In spite of the fact that you say "I don't understand this mindfulness thing," the thing you must realize is that you're already practicing it, but you don't know it. Mindfulness is at your disposal whenever you wish to use it, however it requires discipline to use its benefits effectively.

The Origin of Mindfulness

Since 1970, psychiatry as well as child psychology have used mindfulness in various treatments. Mindfulness is a concept that has its roots in Buddhism as well as Hinduism. Mindfulness is "Smrti," in Sanskrit meaning to keep in mind, remember or to remember. In the Vedas which are the oldest texts in Hinduism it is given the title "Sati" which means to recall. The idea came from the East and then spread to the West and was extremely well-known.

In Hinduism mindfulness is practiced as a part of Vedic meditation. Hinduism and Buddhism have many similarities. In Buddhism the path to awakening is heavily influenced by mindfulness. Sati or mindfulness is believed to be as the first step towards attaining the path of enlightenment. Both of them are based by dharma, a concept that seeks to bring people to a harmonious relationship with world.

Jon KabatZinn is the person responsible for Jon Kabat-Zinn is responsible for bringing mindfulness to his home in the East into the West by establishing the Center for Mindfulness at the University of Massachusetts Medical School. He also created a center at the university, dubbed The Mindfulness-Based Professional Education and Training, which runs an eight-week course to deal with stress. The Mindfulness-Based Stress Reduction Program is well-known. Kabat-Zinn is a Buddhist. Buddhist roots and was able to successfully integrate his Eastern roots in Western science.

Despite its religious roots It does not require that one be religious in order to be mindful. It is a mindset which can be learned and developed so that people can be capable of gaining its advantages. Over time it has been proved effective in relieving symptoms of depression, stress addiction, stress, and psychosis. These programs are being implemented in prisons, hospitals, veterans centers schools, as well as other institutions.

Why Should You Live in the Present?

The term mindfulness can be described in various ways, but it's basically, "Living in the moment." It's about the ability to let go about the past and the future in order to live the present moment as it unfolds. It's crucial as it allows you to appreciate life more. When you are in the present you are able to be present in every aspect of life and you are able to enjoy everything. If you're in the present and fully present, you don't lose the chance to live your life.

Are you caught your past? Perhaps you've experienced traumatizing events, and can't let go of the events that took place. It is possible that the past has done this to people, however this desire to dwell on the past is useless since there is no way you can ever going to be able to restore the past. This is also true of worrying too much regarding the future. If you're worried about managing things to ensure that you are in control of the events that will occur in the next few days, weeks, months or even decades in the future, you miss out on the chance to watch things happen as they ought to.

Are you so concerned about the future and the past? Do you not realize that you're not able to live your life in the present because you're looking elsewhere? You must remain present as your life is nothing in the event that you don't do what you are supposed to. So, it doesn't matter whether things are going well or badly and you must live your life to the fullest.

Debunking Mindfulness Myths

Before you get in the text, it's important to clear any doubts you might have regarding mindfulness. There are many myths surrounding mindfulness. They stem from misinformation, therefore the solution to this lies is to set the record truthful.

What are some myths that must be spelled out?

Mindfulness was not created to help you fix your. Perhaps you're feeling that your life is chaotic and you're in need of a shift. Mindfulness isn't a magic solution to problems. Mindfulness will not help you to get back on track to allow you to live the best life. It's just an attitude that helps you have a better grasp of the events that are taking place.

Mindfulness is not a way to help you avoid reality. Many people believe that meditation and mindfulness are about escaping reality. through focusing on the distraction and focusing on the present, you train your mind to be able to focus on the present and not worry about reality. Mindfulness isn't about escape. It is more about returning to ensure that you don't lose yourself in.

Mindfulness does not mean getting rid of your thoughts. Because it's not a way to escape, it permits the mind to be occupied. It's not easy to eliminate thoughts from your brain particularly when you are struggling by things. Mindfulness is not a way to require you to end your thoughts. Instead, it trains you to regain your focus, regardless of the noise your thoughts make.

The practice of mindfulness is not a cure. There is nothing miraculous about what mindfulness can do, however, those who have the greatest success with this belief have noticed a shift in their lives that merits admiration. Many people believe they have found an ultimate "cure all" for all sorts of ailments however it's not. It's simply an attitude that changes the way your brain functions to are more effective. And if it is successful in solving the issue, it's awe-inspiring.

It is not an actual religion. As mentioned previously the practice of mindfulness has a religious origins, but it doesn't necessarily belong to any particular faith. The practices of mindfulness may appear religious, however it's a state of mental state that creates a sense of peace that mimics the religious and that's it. You don't have to be religious to engage in mindfulness. You can not be a part of an affiliation with a religion, but still follow this method.

What made you decide to pick up this book? Do you feel like you're losing control? Are you constantly struggling with the noises that are coming from your head, from the people around you and from the outside and don't know what to do? Mindfulness isn't the solution however it can assist you in finding solutions to your life's difficulties. It can help bring your mind back to the state of peace which helps you be more in control of the circumstances.

You bought this book because you wanted to be in control, and to be able to change your mind at will.

Chapter 1: What Is Social Anxiety?

Have you ever had the pleasure of being a wallflower?

In the days of middle school proms and dances at high school there was no huge thing. If you're feeling uneasy or sweaty and uncomfortable at social gatherings, such as dinners and parties, or discussions, or gatherings, you may be suffering from social anxiety.

Here's a quick test to help you figure out whether you're doing:

Do you feel you are extremely shy or uncomfortable at social settings?

Are you finding it difficult to be a part of team efforts or work in groups due to your shyness?

Do you shy away from public speaking? Or even one-on-one or group discussions with anyone else than your family members or close acquaintances?

Are you worried about what others consider you when you attend social gatherings? Are you worried about what people think of you at gatherings or events?

Are you concerned that you could make a mistake, be embarrassing, or not be interesting during a talk or a meeting? Are you worried that you might offend someone? to avoid them , or the reason you don't speak?

Are you concerned about being the focal point and being ridiculed or the source of embarrassment, shame or even humiliation?

Are you constantly anxious about other people finding out your anxiety that you don't get to enjoy every social event?

Are you hesitant to meet or speaking to people in authority?

Do you prefer eating by yourself or with a handful of chosen family or friends? Do you prefer to refrain from sharing tables or eating out in public?

Are you described as a quiet person or quiet person? Or the shy type?

If you answered the majority or each of those questions a 'yes then you could be saying that you suffer from symptoms that are a result of social anxiety or extreme shyness. The condition of being shy is common particularly when you are confronted by strangers, however many people can manage it. Other social gatherings like black tie events or those attended by celebrities who are above average are likely to trigger timidity or shyness, but it isn't enough to be counted as signs of anxiety in social situations.

However, extreme shyness could be described as an increased sense of anxiety for those who choose to avoid social and public gatherings. If that shyness is so extreme that even a normal lunchtime, when no seating or sharing of tables is necessary is a stressful experience. If the discomfort or distress is extending to other events such as individual discussions, group gatherings or after-work gatherings, you might suspect the shyness is a different issue. If you are unable to lead a happy life, pursue the activities you love doing, or are confident enough to attend the school or workplace or go to work, you might are suffering from a social anxiety disorder.

It is believed that the National Institute for Mental Health classified Social anxiety as an illness, or social phobia, if the sufferer has a severe fear of being judged and/or humiliated or criticised by others until it affects their daily interactions in addition to the capability to form friendships and socialize. Of course, everyone can be uncomfortable, nervous or scared to speak to authorities when they attend a party, or speak to the crowd. But people who suffer from social anxiety disorder have trouble even prior to the event and even in everyday settings like speaking to managers or supervisors when eating at the restaurant, going to an event in public or taking part in a discussion group. They have rapid heartbeats with profuse sweating, redness and more anxiety in the stomachs of their.

In this regard there are psychologists who consider excessive shyness, as well as social anxiety as one in the same because the triggers and symptoms for both are the same.

Do you have social anxiety to be worried about?

Many people who are only aware of shyness typically think it's something they can easily to overcome. In the majority of cases, this could be the case. However, people suffering from social anxiety tend to think negatively about themselves, which interferes with treatment. Self-pity, negative thinking or apathy, feelings of inadequateness self-doubt, and incompetence often cause social anxiety.

It is therefore crucial to know what causes it and then stop any further growth of the disorder to obtain a successful as well as permanent cure for the rest of your life.

Chapter 2: Anxiety

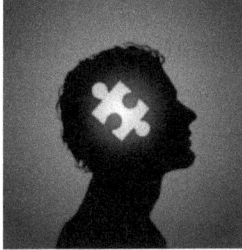

If a person is thinking about "anxiety," often what comes to mind is someone who is constantly worried or has an anxiety-related habit or tick. While these are symptoms that are a result of stress, this kind of disorder can also manifest as symptoms that go beyond the normal level of nervousness. If not treated, certain types of anxiety may go towards hazardous, and can result in suicide or accidental death.

Life is filled with stress, anxiety, stress and sometimes disappointments. It's normal to experience moments of anxiety. However, when the fear or anxiety becomes persistent or apathetic, it has changed from a normal method of self-preservation and protection to an issue that requires care. In the same way, someone may dislike things like the snake or a particular kind of food. However, if the fear becomes a chronic and uncontrollable fear that makes them think of snakes everywhere or gain an eating disorder treatment must be sought out immediately.

What is Anxiety?

Our body, as it is called, is a marvellous body that is capable of carrying out thousands of procedures each minute. While it is believed of the brain being distinct from body functions, current research has proven that there is a direct link between our emotional, mental physical, and mental states. Although stress is a natural aspect of our lives, a persistent lack of ability to handle everyday tensions, or having constant anxiety or stress, could be the sign of a deeper issue.

People who suffer with chronic anxiety suffer anxiety, fear or phobias specific in a way that hinders the ability of them to keep a balanced of functioning and attitude. It could manifest as inability to socialize or interacting with others, a fear of certain items or locations or objects, an emotional reaction to past traumas or an overwhelming anxiety and sadness. There are many types of anxiety that have been recognized and we will discuss the most common areas throughout this course.

What Causes Anxiety?

There are a myriad of variables that could influence the creation of anxiety. Certain of them are biological aspects within us and others external.

Neurotransmitters, chemical messengers, along with hormones make up the elements in the body that affect the state of mind and anxiety. Both transmit brain signals and regulate mental, physical and emotional wellbeing. Any deficiency in these crucial brain chemicals can have the potential to drastically alter mood and affect the capacity of an individual to cope with trauma or stress in a healthy way. This is the reason behind the sudden , or increasingly unpredictable behavior of sufferers of severe depression or anxiety.

Neurotransmitters are chemical signals made by neurons, that travel and attach to the receptors of neurons and cells. Neurotransmitters can be classified in two types: Excitatory neurotransmitters which trigger the neuron cell to activate or to perform an action (example adrenaline) and inhibitory neurotransmitters which trigger the neuron to block the action (example --- serotonin).

If a neurotransmitter is associated with anxiety or uncertain, the brain releases adrenaline, also referred to as epinephrine. It's an endocrine and a neurotransmitter that is affecting almost every body part. Adrenaline is the primary chemical messenger that activates our human body's "fight or flight" mechanism which is activated in the face of danger.

Adrenaline is an effective substance because it helps keep us safe from danger and gives us an additional energy boost to endure difficult situations. In modern times, there's an incessant stream of stimulation, which activates our body's stress reaction, and creates a constant surge of adrenaline. As time passes, a feeling of anxiety, hyperactivity and even paranoia may be the result.

A hormone can also be an organic chemical messenger that moves through the bloodstream , and transmits instructions to different organs and cells, telling them know when to stop, begin or speed up a process. Additionally, they affect emotional and mental balance hormones also regulate appetite and fat storage, sleep as well as other functions. A lack of hormones' ability to function as they should can lead to mental as well as physical ailments that may cause anxiety.

Consider, for instance the hormone called melatonin. The powerful hormone is produced in the pineal gland located inside the brain. Melatonin is the hormone responsible for controlling the body's internal clock and it's biological clock. One of the components is the regulation of the sleep cycle. In the event of an interruption in the production of melatonin it can cause insomnia and then restlessness -which is the inability to sleep even when exhausted. As you can imagine, prolonged lack of sleep can result in extreme irritability, forgetfulness and anxiety.

Alongside the issues with the internal workings that the human body is experiencing, external elementslike trauma, diet, and stress can affect our mood and create the conditions for the creation of anxiety disorders.

Common Types of Anxiety

Anxiety manifests in a variety of kinds However, the most well-known types according to the National Institute for Mental Health include:

* General Anxiety Disorder

* Obsessive Compulsive Disorder (OCD)

* Panic Disorder

* Social Phobia

* Post-traumatic Stress Disorder

Other types of anxiety include agoraphobia separation anxiety, childhood anxiety and a variety of eating disorders. People can develop an anxiety or phobia due to any reason, and may not be listed in the above list. But, in this course, you'll be exposed to a variety of treatments that can be effective in the treatment of most forms of anxiety.

Anxiety Statistics

For many anxiousness is a real and uncomfortable aspect of life. Anxiety affects everyone regardless of race or age situation. The National Institute for Mental Health In 2005, about 18.5% of the US population was suffering from anxiety disorders. In those cases 23, percent (or 4 percent) from the US population were classified as having severe. The number is likely to have increased in the past few years and shows that Americans require more assistance in the prevention and management of anxiety.

Furthermore, women are also more likely to be suffering from anxiety. Studies have shown that women are 60% more likely to develop anxiety disorders in their lives than males. Additionally the white population is twenty percent more likely suffer from anxiety than blacks while 30 percent higher to suffer from anxiety than Hispanics. The typical time to experience anxiety in America is 11 years old and this is a huge concern.

Based on the information above, anxiety poses a real danger to the wellbeing and health many millions. However, by making lifestyle changes, discovering ways to manage anxiety, and applying proven treatment methods anxiety can be managed and even reversed.

Chapter 3: How I Overcame Anxiety: A Personal Story

It's difficult to remember the exact moment when my anxiety journey began. Since a very early age, I was worried about the actions of other people and I can clearly recall feeling very unsure because I would constantly be thinking about what others were thinking of me. The truth is, I was not the most popular student at school. My family was 30 miles from any city in the town I was in. Therefore, I never ever had the opportunity to have time with my peers of older than the classroom. I did not have a close connection with my peers. I did have "friends" but as we became older and high school began, I didn't belong to any group of social people. If I was noticed by the crowd that was popular the majority of them knew that I was smart, and was a good student and copied my. If I was noticed by those who were jocks it was because of an favor. If the outcasts threw a punch at me the reason was to keep things that weren't to be carried into school with my backpack. In truth, I was an unwelcome visitor. My only goal was be somewhere , and to be human not a person who was deemed to be important to anyone. Anyone.

Growing up was not easy. I was rejected, ostracized and bullied simply because no one took the time to learn about me. I was viewed as different due to the fact that although my mind was flooded with thoughts and ideas I was unable to let my anxiety leave an envelop over my mouth, making me afraid to speak my mind. I was always trapped in my shell and nervous to let my personal colors shine. I'm not saying that it wasn't a problem sometimes, I had some amazing breaks. I had a good friend or two who were nice to my personality for what it was. However, school was not the one where I felt secure. I was more comfortable writing my thoughts about people out on my bedroom. Whatever I did, no matter how many times I swooned individuals or attempted to establish relationships, I didn't succeed. I never was the girl chosen for prom and was never the first choice when it came to sports. If I was involved with other school events, it was not visible to those around me. I am convinced that what happened during my time in high school, when my hormones were raging was the time when anxiety took up a space in my life, which no one could fill.

My childhood was nothing but awful although my family struggled frequently. They gave both my sister and me with everything that we required to live. However, I would like to have provided us with more opportunities to live the world beyond school. There were no sleepovers or even had the chance to be a part of a sleepover. We were never able to meet people after school, as we would have to hop onto the bus to catch a ride straight to our homes. What made my becoming so dark was my lack of connection with other people and the feeling of being alone. I was constantly feeling like my voice was snatched away. I was afraid to speak out, afraid of having my ideas smacked back. I would cry myself to sleep often, because I was required to go to a location each day where I was not loved or accepted. It was as if I had the option of visiting prison, but with a slender death sentence in one, not exactly joyful bundle.

My anxiety prevented me from speaking my unique voice in front of my class. In the instances where I had the opportunity to perform before a crowd of my classmates and teachers, negativity flooded my mind and my confidence waned. I became the odd child who didn't care about it, since there were many days in which I was physically present, but not mentally or emotionally. When I saw my friends develop bonds and keep them with each other however, I was the girl who eventually became content in my own space, writing in my journal at lunchtime. I believe to some, I was referred to for being the "writing girl." I needed to. My raging anxious thoughts would always overwhelm my little jolly feelings that I was able to experience on occasions. On paper, anyone would likely think I was an expert. However, as it turned out I graduated from high school in a way that was unnoticeable, even with the prizes I won through my writing kindness to others, and dedication to the classroom.

Then , college came around. I was far from my comfortable zone. I was far from my comfort zone. I was in the dorm with three roommates during my first year at college. I was terrified to death. I didn't know what to do, how to do, or even what. The confusion revealed the most dreaded parts of anxiety. From literally pulling my hair to anxious movements, there were many days when I felt like I was overwhelmed. I was unable to keep myself in check and control my physical self. There were many occasions that after class, I spent a large portion the time inside my dorm by myself. I was comfortable in this manner. I was a bit isolated. My anxiety prevented me from functioning as a normal teenager. It seems that people were offended for refusing to accept their invitations.

After that, I began to get to know one of my roommates more. As time passed I broke to terms with my shyness, and soon, we were very good friends. While we weren't at the same level and prestigious school, I eventually got to meet the family members and acquaintances of her, and began to understand what it was like to not be confined by my location. This eased my anxiety a lot by itself. I shared with my friends that I had written some of my writings . And when I was greeted with love back the years of suffering through high school appeared worthy of it.

The following year in college, a lot of my friends from my first year transferred to other schools or left. This forced me to start over. This time, I had the privilege of being a Resident assistant at the dorms that were newer. I made connections easily that were actually meaningful however my anxiety was able to take the best of me on most times. But, I still made lifelong acquaintances that offered me a chance, despite my numerous rants of negative thoughts. It was the same year when I got out of my closet to my friends and family. This added a new dimension in my life which initially made me uncomfortable. As I learned to accept my own self, my friends and other acquaintances accepted my wholeheartedly. I began to feel a sense of love for my self for the very first time in my life.

The following year, I took the police dispatching position which I got through a friend of mine who also worked with me. That was when my stress increased to the point that I nearly could not perform my duties properly. Being responsible for lives that required saving was just too for me to handle. The other day, as I was preparing to go to work, I experienced the first panic attack I could not control. It was so intense that I shook for a short time and nearly smashed my car. A night-time stay in the local hospital resulted in therapy and doctor appointments, during which I was diagnosed as having depression anxiety. Let me tell you the truth, getting given Xanax for my condition that was newly discovered proved to be extremely helpful. I was able to control the way I lived my daily life while. However, in spite of the vast amount of knowledge I gained from this job I left with a heavy heart of worry with a constant watching my back to avoid being hit in the back once more. I decided to move in with the people I made at college in a town that was about half an hour's drive away.

A new city forced me with the task of starting from scratch once more, but I am happy that, since then, I've always had strong trust relationships to help me stay grounded. When I was juggling jobs and moved to various homes with friends during the course of two years I finally reached out for assistance, but to much effect. The therapist I had been seeing? When I finally had the courage to share my emotions and my tiniest thoughts which I'd kept within me for the span of my life I was able to see her fall in bed with me. Yes, my therapist whom I paid an amount of money to, fell asleep while I was speaking. I left the room without a glimmer of faith in humanity. If someone hired to listen and assist me was unable to help me I was devastated. Suicide thoughts were a constant thought. Thankfully, I didn't have an incredibly strong heart to cut myself off to my friends and relatives who really love me. It was during my lowest points when I realized that I needed to decide for myself to take matters into my hands, and stop relying on others to support me in my mental state.

I realized that I had missed from a large portion of the youthful portion of my life. I decided I had to take control of my life in order not to sink so deeply that I would be unable to get myself out of the mess I was becoming. I had grown tired of living at a distance from people in the dark of my bedroom, surrounded by only my thoughts and emotions. I realized that nobody would want to be constantly with people who behaved the way I did. I let anxiety rule my life. There was no one situation that triggered a light bulb in my brain telling me that I needed to make a change. It was a series of years of experiences which anxiety had forced me through until I decided it was time to stop.

It didn't happen in a flash, but when I began writing again and read other stories of people's lives I learned some methods I would never think of trying. As a young person, I did not just find myself back however, by using a variety of strategies in general I was able to keep track of my own anxiety disorders by only taking medication only when absolutely necessary. It has completely changed my life, which can be the main reason why I'm happy to share my successes with you!

When you go through the subsequent chapters, the title suggests, there are 10 simple ways to ease anxiety and avoid panic attacks as well as other dreadful signs of anxiety. There are more than 10 methods covered in this book, those that are listed 1-10 are the ones I have found the most beneficial and helped me on a path to happiness in my personal life. I would suggest that you try the strategies that are listed first however, I am not here to instruct you on what you should do with your life! If you find a method that you like or something you'd like to try at all times you should not be hesitant.

This book stands out from the rest. Instead of being a collection of academic jargon I'm here to address the serious mental illness that affects people who suffer from it or have friends or family members who are suffering from anxiety in a personal manner. When you are turning the page I'm trying to remind you you're not the only one suffering from anxiety and that there are some things you can start to incorporate into your daily life today, to get you out from the hole that anxiety could have pushed you into. Best of luck as you go through the rest of the sections with me. I hope that you will find at least a little glimmer of hope in the pages ahead.

Chapter 4: Why Is Confidence Important For Your Professional Life?

Mastering Confidence in Your Conversations

Effectively communicating your thoughts, feelings concerns, wishes, and desires is vital in any relationship, not just your professional relationships. We'll go over how it can impact romantic relationships in the future.

The ability to communicate effectively can boost your confidence as the ability to communicate with others can make you feel intelligent and at ease, loved and engaged. Have you noticed the way you feel when you aren't able to convey your thoughts? Perhaps your mind is more quickly than you speak, or perhaps you're not able to come up with the right word or expression. It's an unpleasant feeling that may leave us feeling somewhat deflated and small.

If you'd like to feel confident in your speaking skills, Try these strategies. Introduce them gradually into your daily routine gradually, one at a time. Once you've got it down you can move onto the next. If one of them doesn't work for you, leave it out and go to a different one. You can always return to it in the future and test it out again.

Prepare yourself.

One of the reasons that some conversations are a mess is that either or both parties weren't completely prepared. Similar to when you are preparing an upcoming presentation, you must know the key aspects you're looking to include and ensure that you are aware of what the topic of your discussion is.

If you are attending an informal luncheon with customers to discuss about a new product you need to market do not enter the discussion without knowing any information about the product. Be prepared for their inquiries by running a brief rundown of questions with a coworker or someone else from the same department, or with a acquaintance.

Furthermore it is also a good idea to prepare talk points in case there's an absence of conversation. The best way to accomplish this is to ensure that you're up-to-date with the latest news. If you're not able to sit and watch a newscast early in the day, glance through the newsfeed on the search engine, or your social media feeds or even apps on your smartphone.

Be aware of what you would like from an interaction

In professional interactions, you don't often have luncheons to have a social gathering without any agenda. Sure, there's an objective behind these lunches, but it's usually not simply "to catch up".

Even if you did not invite this discussion, you may still have a need or desired outcome from this discussion. If you are aware of the outcome you're seeking and you know where you'd like it to go to , and you'll be more precise with your responses. There'll be less sputtering and struggling to find the right words which is always a good thing.

Learn how to lead the conversation.

This doesn't mean you have to be able to control conversations. If you have to steer a conversation either way then you must be equipped to be able to do it. The ability to steer the conversation towards an area you know about will do a good amount to boost confidence in the situation as well as with the individual you're talking with.

Depending on the way you approach this, you could be extremely manipulative (we'll be careful not to do this) or you can be subtle and nimble, but also clear.

Be sure to be conscious and engaged during the discussion. This means you're actually listening (not pretending to be listening while you're really creating your response in your mind).

Answer any questions or statements and don't respond to them. It's a good idea to do this regardless of the conversation you're in, but it's often neglected. If you respond to comments or questions, you're typically preoccupied with what you desire and this can result in a rapid increase in the tone and anger. If you react to someone else, you are paying attention, pondering your the logic behind your response, and you are refusing for self-defense and "be right".

Inquire and Validate. You can ask them about themselves and the reasons for their beliefs. Be sure to confirm their motives and beliefs as well.

Declare your intentions. Reorient the conversation through stating positive intent to the conversation. "My intention wasn't for it to devolve into a screaming match but to calmly exchange ideas in order to make the best decision for the company and for this project."

Reschedule. The purpose for redirecting conversation should be to shift towards a direction that is more productive , if needed. If you cannot redirect it in this manner, you might have to schedule an alternative time. This is fine as long as you are able to catch it in time (without excessively heated remarks or declarations) and you're courteous when you announce your intentions.

Be grateful for the exchange. It's not that you have to thank the person for their time, but "thank you for talking to me" but thanking someone for a productive discussion, an open mind, or even the time, honesty, and willingness to consider your viewpoint is essential. This opens the door for greater dialogue in the future.

Chapter 5: Healthy Diet, Healthy Body And Healthy Mind

The majority of anxiety disorders have been thought of as mental disorders, and the connection to general health and nutrition are only just beginning to be established. But, in the present, doctors and psychologists are starting to look at the complicated relationship between how your brain functions as well as the way their function is affected by the diet we eat and our exercise.

It might seem unlikely that food choices affect your mood, but think about the simple case of caffeine. We all know that if we require a boost in energy or concentration, then caffeine is the most efficient route for both! The brains of our bodies are, at the end of the day, just organs in the body. The energy we supply to them (and the way that energy is delivered in) could have a significant impact on the brain's chemical chemistry and, in turn, influence our mood.

In this section we'll look at ways to increase your mood, lessen anxiety attacks, and lead an enjoyable and healthy life. These two methods aren't "quick fixes" but as you incorporate them into your daily routine, you'll find that the frequency and intensity of anxiety attacks will be dramatically decreased. Think of these strategies as "slow-burners", which will aid you in dealing with anxiety-related issues over the long term.

Technique # 1 Anxiety Dieting

This isn't the latest diet trend to shed weight! Dieting to reduce anxiety is all about eating healthy. As we've mentioned eating the foods we eat can have an immediate (often quick-acting) influence on our mood as well as our emotional state. A healthy, balanced diet is not only essential for good physical health an ideal weight that is stable and healthy is also essential for your mental well-being.

A healthy diet should contain an equal amount of these foods:

Protein sources that are low-fat (lean meat, pulses and/or apricots)

A wide variety of fruits and vegetables

Complex carbs (whole grain cereals, pasta and breads) but if you'd prefer gluten-free slow carbs, you can try lentils, beans, leafy vegetables (broccoli as well as spinach is both highly suggested) Oatmeal sweet potatoes, brown rice.

Fish oily (mackerel as well tuna)

There are many types of food which you might need to stay clear of in case you suffer with anxiety.

Foods high in sugar, they increase our energy levels rapidly However, they may also increase adrenaline production, which can cause anxiety.

Processed food items; they often contain high levels sugar, as well as other additives that can alter the chemical balance within your brain, which can lead to more or worse panic attacks.

Caffeine: as stated above caffeine can give you an energy boost, and a cup is generally fine. But, if you drink too much it can trigger chemical imbalances in your brain that over-stimulate adrenaline production increasing stress levels.

The long-term use of alcohol may cause anxiety disorders to develop. This is often a sign of the condition and people suffering from depression-related ailments. Eliminating alcohol consumption is highly recommended , however seeking assistance in this regard is sensible.

Certain foods are more beneficial to us in comparison to others. When you think about brain food particular foods can have a profound effects in our mental state. The following foods have been proven to have positive effects on brain functioning and chemical processes. If you suffer from anxiety-related issues, including them in your diet is essential.

Complex Carbohydrates (mentioned in the previous paragraph) can affect the amount of serotonin the brain produces. It is among our naturally produced "happy" drugs. The increase in serotonin production could help reduce anxiety and depression. The foods that fall into this category are baked potatoes, whole grain wheats and whole-grain pastas, as well as oatmeal-based cereal products.

Vitamin B is crucial to maintain good physical health. it helps manage mood. Vitamin supplements are a good source, including citrus fruits as well as leafy green veggies, chicken eggs, and eggs.

Another important ingredient is Omega-3 as Vitamin B aids to control mood and offers a range of physical benefits. It is found in oily fish such as mackerel, herring and salmon and Sardines. As part of a balanced diet, it is recommended at eating at least two or three portions each week.

Technique #2 Exercise and Anxiety

If the thought of going to the gym can cause panic attacks It's likely that you're not the only one. You don't have to be suffering from social anxiety (or any other anxiety-related disorder) to be averse to going to the gym! But healthy exercise can have many surprising consequences for those suffering from anxiety disorders as well as other psychological disorders like depression. The mechanisms that physical exercise and psychological health interact aren't fully known, however many medical professionals around the world recognize that exercise has significant effects on a variety of psychological disorders. It's even believed that exercise is as effective in battling depression as a variety of commonly prescribed medications.

Here's the good news There is absolutely no requirement to join an exercise class. If you're interested, there's absolutely no harm signing up. But, "exercise", in this case, is a reference to simple, simple exercises that anyone can manage. In short, brief bursts of activity couple of times per day is the kind of exercise experts suggest. A strenuous walk that lasts only 10 minutes is thought to to raise your mood for several hours. For people suffering from anxious disorders, it might be difficult to get out and about every now and then. For those suffering from severe issues, it might seem like a nightmare. But, exercising can aid in improving your mental health and relieve your mind of stress. Utilize the tips below to boost the chances of being able to incorporate fitness into your routine.

Do not start with the goal of running 10 miles. Instead, focus on small bursts exercise - that will leave you exhausted and sweating throughout the day. 10 minutes each time is more than a half hour all in one go.

Moderate-intensity exercises are recommended to improve your physical health as well as your mental health. This means walking fast biking, jogging, cycling or swimming. Jogging and walking do not require any investments and if you're not comfortable alone, join a group with a friend or a relative. You should try to connect with someone who's dealing with the same issues , or has a solid understanding of these issues for additional assistance.

Psychologists suggest that the exercise you select should be regular and repetitive. This helps to clear your mind and helps focus it on the task at your hands. Walking is the easiest of them all and is likely to be simple to accomplish for most people.

If you notice that you are experiencing anxiety after a certain period of exercise , simply concentrate your attention upon your breathing. Utilize a technique of meditation such as "mindfulness meditation" (described briefly in the following chapter) to be aware of your bodyand your breathing, and to reduce the effect of thoughts that are negative or anxious. Be aware of the present moment it is, rather than the thoughts which are in your head. Alternately, take a step at a time (out-loud in case it is required) to disengage your mind from feelings of fear.

Chapter 6: Identifying Stressors

Recognizing the triggers that cause stress within your own life can be the very first thing you do to decreasing the amount of stress you experience. Every person is affected by stressors in a different way, so the fact that something can be stressful for one person , it does not mean it's going to be a burden for you. This means that even if something causes stress to you, others might not be able to comprehend because it's not something they can relate to.

Certain stressors are easy to spot. For instance, getting late to work, forgetting you'd had an appointment or being trapped in traffic. Sometimes, it's the smallest things we never think about.

Remember that it's not just bad things that can create stress. Things that are good can cause stress. It doesn't mean you have to quit doing them. This means you must to be able to identify when stress reaches a point that you require action to alleviate it.

An excellent illustration of a positive thing that could trigger stress is:

You're helping a friend with her wedding which is scheduled to take place in two weeks. You are obviously thrilled because she's planning to get married and you'd like to be a part of the process. But it can be stressful on you due to time constraints or having to re-arrange your timetable.

The things that make us feel stressed aren't good for us. If you know immediately what they are can be, here are some indicators to look for.

Inability to take simple choices.

Forgetfulness.

Distracted easily.

Over-thinking and worrying.

The tendency to look at everything in a negative light.

Anxiety or depression.

Low self-confidence or self-esteem.

Insufficiency of motivation.

Irritability.

Mood changes.

Panic strikes.

Tired even though you've had enough.

Feeling easily angry or frustrated.

There are many more signs or signs of stress but the ones listed above are an excellent place to begin. If you experience one or more of the symptoms listed above, and you can trace them back to the time they first began, you'll be able to begin to determine what is causing your stress. If you are unable to identify the exact cause but you are able to pinpoint an approximate time frame of events that took place. It could have been an array of events that took place at similar times. There doesn't need to be a single thing. Sometimes, when something goes wrong, all else is just a follow-up. Finding ones stressors are the initial step in attempting to eliminate them.

Chapter 7: I Feel Better...Nevermind!!!! !

Seems crazy, right? Through the years I've been with a myriad of medication and have been to many doctors, each with an opinion on what drugs would be effective for me. I am now a patient that walks into the doctor's office and explains to them all about my medical history, the medicines I've used, what was successful and what didn't. They are always amazed by the level of knowledge I have about my treatment, and how much I have learned about the body.

One thing I've learned from being a person who suffers from depression and anxiety It is that you may not react to the first treatment you test. It's simple and simple...the first batch of medication I tried had various aspects to my body but none of which made me feel as an ordinary person. (What exactly is normal?) The adverse effects made me think about giving the world If depression didn't already put me on the edge. I was clenching my teeth throughout the day, which led to soreness in my jaw and gums. I was starving and was able to go to 140lbs at five' 6 inches to 118 pounds in a matter of months. (I still remember my mom asking me to eat food since my clothing was falling apart and I looked so sick.)

I found a remedy that made me feel happy. I was leading an active lifestyle and eating three large meals per day, as well as snacks. I was a very active, and productive teen. I was in the marching band and the track and field. I also attended honors classes, prepared for college and then graduated as a typical teenager. In this transition to a healthier lifestyle I even ripped apart my favorite pair of pants, which was a clear and funny indication my body was devouring food too much and losing weight. The life was great. (Note That I will avoid mentioning any drug specifically. What I have found to work for me might not be effective for you, and vice to the other. To be as supportive and therapeutic as I can, I will avoid sharing names with you.)

A few years later after having the first of my children, post-partum depression set in, and the medication I was taking already did not work. However much something worked with me, it struggled with the medicine being consistent in long periods of time. The only thing I can say is, take note of your body. Be aware of what feels good and keep that feeling in mind. This will allow you to recognize when you are falling into the dark of depression, even before you're up to your eyes in the darkness. Through my experience of trying various treatments I've come to the conclusion that you must try the most unsuccessful treatments before you get to the golden egg, even if it lasts for a few years. This could include including therapy or counseling as well as adjusting dosages or even changing the medication altogether. Imagine that the goal is to help you achieve the blissful sensation.

If you locate it, you'll be able to feel as if you've lived in darkness all of your life. Then suddenly, the light comes on your life, and you can see things in a more clear and new perspective. Do not let go of the feeling...it is a great feeling and well worth trying to chase.

Chapter 8: How To Deal With Anxiety

In the present at the moment, there are more than 40 million Americans suffering from a form of anxiety or panic attacks. The most common factor is the price dependent on one's life style. Other countries also have high levels of sufferers, too. If you weren't aware of more, you may believe that a global epidemic is taking hold.

Next time, pay careful focus on your behavior when you are arguing with your spouse. Are you having more arguments now than it was before? Do you feel like you are being more cautious about social occasions than you used to? Or are you experiencing fears that seem unreal or fearful? If so, these could be indicators that you're suffering from some kind that is a form of anxiety disorder. There's no doubt that you've experienced the phrase "panic attack." The reality is that they're real, and deadly But remember that there are a variety of anxiety disorders, some are less serious than others.

There's a myth that surrounds anxiety that having an anxiety condition in some way can make one look weak or a negative person to other people. The reality is that there's no person who lives their life without experiencing some kind of anxiety or anxiety at some point or other time.

It's how someone deals with their unrealistic feelings that determines the extent to which they are affecting your life. In a growing segment of society the constant affliction of anxiety is real and there's no evidence of the number of sufferers who remain unreported.

However, what's even more important is that more youngsters and teens are becoming prone to stress and anxiety.

How your body responds to stress is vital to how one can protect themselves from what appears to be dangers. This is an assessment of the likelihood of survival in the face of an event that could be dangerous or in danger itself. The individual's response will vary who is at risk, he/she may either be able to take the pressure by the drum and defend themselves, or withdraw and flee.

The"fight or flight" strategy is the way a person goes about responding to stressful situations regardless of having an emotional trauma in their life. The reactions or choices are a natural fight to survive in everyday interactions. That's why you flip a switch and is either taking the flight or fight approach when you come face with an ensuing danger.

The smell of danger can cause an adrenaline rush in your veins and make your heart beat faster. This can cause you to feel like you're about to faint or weaken. However, the interesting result of this is that the body's prepping you for fight or flight and you can try exercise to combat this sensation.

For the second chances are you'll be surprised by the speed you're able to go! If you are in the phase of fight or flight there are two choices to choose from: 1.) You can be inactive and retreat. 2) You can be aggressive and takes on the threat head-on. If you let yourself allow yourself to be vulnerable to fighting or flight situations frequently and regularly, you could be in danger when you are confronted with dangerous and stressful situations. This eventually can endanger your health.

However, it does not mean that it should influence your life. In the event that you are or someone else you know has suffered from persistent symptoms, such as anxiety or anxiety over the unexpected Now is the time to take a step back to look at your life. The best way to handle anxiety attacks is to control and get rid of it!

What Helps Anxiety - 2 Secrets That Work

If you come facing the challenge of a circumstance, it's normal to be nervous. But, if your anxieties and anxieties affect your daily life and consume you it is possible that you suffer from Anxiety disorders. When your levels of anxiety are over the roof, you might be wondering what causes anxiety. But, only you can assist yourself in cutting your anxiety at the source. You can, however, get your life in order and take back the control over your life making the right choices.

1. Challenge Negative Thoughts

Be open to uncertainty. The fact is that life does not be predictable if you be concerned about every possibility which could happen. you'll stop yourself from enjoying the wonderful things that are happening right now throughout your day. Accept the fact that the future isn't certain and don't look for quick solutions to problems that arise in life. If you're frequently wondering what can provide in easing anxiety, you can spend a particular portion of your day to worrying thoughts.

Make a time for worry Make a time in your day to completely devoted to anxiety. This will be your anxiety time, and you will be able to focus solely on negative, anxious thoughts in that moment and not try to fix them. Be sure to not get stressed throughout the remainder of the day. You can note down any thoughts of anxiety that pop into your mind, and you can concentrate on them throughout your worrying time.

Note down your thoughts that cause anxiety whenever you feel stressed write down your thoughts that cause anxiety on a piece of paper, or write it down on your smartphone or laptop. Not just can the act of writing down your anxiety-inducing thoughts distract you from them and eliminate them however, you may be able to focus on thinking about them in the future, after your anxiety-related time in the event that you choose to.

2. Take Care of Yourself

Make a conscious effort to eat healthy: Breakfast is the primary food you eat Therefore, ensure that you start your day by eating a nutritious breakfast and then eat regular smaller, healthy meals throughout the day. Your blood sugar levels could drop if skip meals for too long and you'll be more stressed due to this.

Regular exercise is a proven anxiety-buster and stress reducer. Most days, you should spend at least 30 minutes engage in aerobic exercise if wish to maximize your advantages.

Make sure you get enough sleep. Sleep deprivation can increase your anxiety and thoughts, therefore you must try to sleep at least 7-8 hours of restful nighttime sleep, as this is among the most important factors that aids in reducing anxiety.

Relaxation techniques to practice If you regularly practice relaxation techniques like deep breaths or mindfulness meditation as well as progressive relaxation of muscles consistently it can improve your the sense of well-being and emotional calm while also reducing the symptoms of anxiety.

Beware of smoking and drinking alcohol. It's a common misconception that smoking cigarettes or drinking alcohol can help relieve your anxieties and worries however, an excessive intake of either could cause greater anxiety.

Anxiety is a normal reaction of our body however if your stress makes you think about what causes anxiety relief you should consider the following steps can help to reduce your anxiety with time.

Affirmations for Anxiety and How to Use Them

Affirmations for anxiety are phrases which can assist you in reducing signs of anxiety. These affirmations are great uplifting ideas that you can use frequently to lessen the chances of suffering the anxiety-related attack. It is also possible to use these affirmations to help you fight the anxiety attacks or issues that will not disappear with time. The battle against panic attacks requires a determination and positive affirmations for panic will boost your ability to resist such attacks, so that your mind will be at ease at times when it is necessary. By using these affirmations, you will see positive results in overcoming anxiety attacks.

There are a myriad of in affirmations for anxiety. Everyone suffers from different kinds of attack and it's up to them to locate the right words to calm their minds and help them get away from the attacks. The whole process is based on changing negative thoughts into positive ones and is the sole non-medicated treatment for such ailments. Yes, you can combat anxiety by taking prescribed medications However, as time passes, it can have a negative impact on your health, and the dose will increase with the the passing of time.

Anxiety-related affirmations shouldn't always be used in the midst of an attack. They can be used on a regular basis to change the negative thoughts you're having to positive and constructive ones. People also utilize other techniques such as yoga, deep breathing, and meditation to help with these affirmations to make them stronger and eliminate signs. Here are some helpful suggestions to make affirmations more effective:

Utilize more than one affirmation such as music or an picture of your preferred location. Videos can be extremely helpful with soothing music and pictures of nature and wildlife or any other thing that make you feel happy even in your daily routine.

You could also make a recording of your most popular affirmations and use them in an attack. Focus on the words, and soon your mind will be at an end. A number of psychiatrists recommend that people make use of recorded statements on a every day, even during the ordinary days.

Use your favorite affirmations with the people who know you well. They can calm you by repeating these affirmations prior to or following an attack.

Avoid working with ones that aren't appropriate for you. Everyone is different and may have various symptoms and conditions that could create an attack. Look at your own words. Explore your soul and think about what is it that makes you feel happy.

Affirmations aren't the only solution to anxiety, but if they are practiced regularly they are sure to put you in a better place and help reduce the number of attacks drastically and also reduce the time between attacks. The method is recommended by psychiatrists and doctors for patients suffering from serious psychological and anxiety disorders.

Chapter 9: What Really Is Anxiety?

To fully comprehend anxiety, it is essential to examine the definition of anxiety and what it's not. The primary difference between anxiety and fear is that the fear you experience is usually attributed to a particular situation or object. Fear is a genuine relationship with your nervous system, which your brain has learned over time. The fear usually refers to something that is likely to happen. taking place. You may be worried about that your partner will leave you and not showing up on time for work, or being physically assaulted and running out of money or being verbally abused by someone close to. If you are experiencing anxiety, in contrast, it could be very difficult to pinpoint the precise cause. A lot of my patients have admitted to me that they were suffering from multiple phobias but in reality they were suffering from anxiety.

As the anxiety diminished, as did the feelings related to the phobias. There was no any specific treatment directed at the phobias in themselves. The feeling of anxiety is more personal than external. It can be frustratingly incomprehensible, confusing, or disorienting. Our thoughts are often not believed, when we are suffering from anxiety, many of the explanations and assumptions they formulate will be wrong. However, after a few months or years, they could be very actual to the person you are, as they might feel real emotionally. True however they're not the issue, and it's an unnecessary use of your energy, your emotions, and time exploring them in search of the answers, but often, they are leading you in the wrong direction.

If your fear is an eerie feeling it is a feeling that "something is wrong" or the fear of "losing control" or "being discovered or caught out" it is important to realize that knowing the specific significance or cause of anxiety isn't necessary to be free from anxiety.

Anxiety can take over your whole existence!

It's a massive reaction of your psychology, physiology and behaviour patterns all simultaneously. On a physiological level anxiety can manifest as a fast heartbeat sweating, dry mouth, the twitching. On a psychological scale, it may create tension in your nervous system , which can hinder the ability of you to control your behavior, remain the "normal" self and complete your normal daily tasks. Psychologically speaking, anxiety can cause an uneasy feeling and fear. Some people even experience creating a sense of separation from the world, and the fear of death or becoming insane.

A lot of people who are diagnosed as depressed, phobic or bipolar actually suffer from anxiety in the majority of cases, and once the anxiety has been removed, all of the other ailments have been eliminated. Anxiety is a cause or trigger of a myriad of emotional, mental and behavioral issues. Many people try to treat the mental and emotional problems without first understanding anxiety as the glue that holds all the patterns. If you can eliminate anxiety first, other issues will be eliminated. their intensity, speed and influence over you. You'll find yourself having a sense of stability in your emotions and capable of moving forward in your life independently. The gruelling mental and emotional attack that anxiety can trigger will go away and you will be able to live your life without the necessity of psychologists, doctors or therapists as a perpetual way to get around.

You will be able to rely on yourself since you'll take charge of your life!

The fact that anxiety isn't "all in your head" is vital when choosing the most effective method to take in the direction you want to go. Anxiety impacts the body on a physiological as well as a psychological and behavioural level. It must be acknowledged for any long-lasting peace. An absolute and permanent relief from anxiety is only accomplished when we are able to intervene at all levels of the three to

Annihilate avoidance behavior

Reduce the physiological Reactivity

Alter the subconscious and conscious beliefs that keep you in an uneasy state and anxiety. (the limitation of beliefs, associations and rationalizations, the concentration of the mind, and the disempowering internal dialogue)

Most people experience anxiety. It isn't a straightforward and regular issue. It can manifest in a variety of diverse forms with various levels of severity. It could vary from a nagging sensation of unease to a frightening panic attack. An anxiety that doesn't appear to be triggered by any particular event or stimulus is known as "free floating anxiety" which is, in its most extreme form, is a panic attack. If anxiety is only triggered due to a particular circumstance, it's called"phobic anxiety" or situational anxiety. Situational anxiety is different from everyday anxieties because it's often unfounded, incompatible or excessive. If you feel a significant fear of driving on roads that you do not know, talking to strangers, or even facing your boss at work, it might be the case.

Situational anxiety is only fearful when you decide trying to escape the circumstance. This could happen when you abandon taking new roads or talking to strangers, and telling your boss the truth completely. Also, phobic anxiety will only occur when you adopt the "strategy of avoidance" from stressful situations. This avoidance behavior is a positive way of reducing discomfort.

In the present, but in the medium to long-term, it can cause an increase in the intensity and frequency of anxiety.

Phobic anxiety happens when a person combines a constant avoidance behavior with a specific fear of the situation, which produces a phobic response. When the pattern develops and continues to grow, the intense anxious feelings may result from only contemplating the specific situation. An individual's anxiety has taken an abrupt shift away from the actual situation, triggering an intense anxiety response until now, it is only thoughts of that scenario turning into a powerful trigger that triggers the intense anxious feeling. This could not happen without the dreadful pattern of avoidance gaining traction.

Imagine that there were 100 people who had an emotional shock of an accident on the train. 50 of them experienced anxiety in the face of a situation, which eventually turned into anxious, while fifty of them continued to suffer without any long-term effects. The primary difference in the way people behave between these two groups is likely to refer to that of the "strategy of avoidance". While it wouldn't stop there, a lot of the 50 individuals who were phobic eventually begin to avoid future circumstances like vehicles, buses or any other place they felt uncontrollable or out of control. The result could be in certain cases to a total refusal to leave their house (agoraphobia). Phobic anxiety could have affected their lives mostly due to being involved in an avoidance pattern. It's the distinction that is the key to the difference. I often see clients who have been following the "strategy of avoidance" for 10, 20 , or up to 50 years. One of the principal assumptions that

The reason I have remained in the position of always stay clear of situations is the belief that I'll be able to put off action until I am more confident in the future.

"The best time to plant a tree was 20 years ago the second best time is today"

The notion that one can be patiently waiting for the perfect moment to confront their fears is extremely risky The ideal time is a figment of imagination that cannot be realized since it doesn't exist. However, it is one of the main elements that prevents the decision-making process today and can cause the delay of your decision for days or months, weeks, and even years. The best time to gain control of your stress is now the longer you delay.

The more resistant you'll become to change quickly and easily. It is not necessary to take a step that is so away from your comfortable zone that it becomes extremely difficult. Reversing the cycle of avoidance is possible by taking tiny, but crucial actions every day that impact every aspect that you are anxious about. For the majority of people who are able to overcome anxiety this is among the most essential steps every person should undertake.

Anticipatory anxiety is one the most important factors that maintain and strengthens the habit of avoidance. When anxiety is triggered through a single thought about a specific situation and you start to worry over what could happen should you decide to confront the fearsome situation and you're experiencing anxiety that is anticipatory. In the most innocuous forms anticipatory anxiety can appear to be "worrying". Sometimes, however, it can be a serious condition that develops and grow to warrant being referred to as anticipatory anxiety.

The major distinction between panic that is spontaneous (anxiety) as well as anticipatory panic (anxiety) is a key element. Anxiety that arises spontaneously can appear out of nowhere, and then reaches an extreme level quickly before easing off gradually. The peak usually occurs in just five minutes, then an easing period that can last for an hour or more. Anxiety and fear can increase in intensity in response to an event or is in panic by worrying about something for a period of time, usually up to an hour. The anxiety usually dissipates quickly when your mind is busy its attention with other things.

Chapter 10: Dealing With Panic Attacks

A major and destructive reactions to anxiety is panic attacks. When you experience this type of reaction, you act out in a bizarre manner. The attack can occur at any time and last for a few minutes. An attack of panic isn't thought of as an individual disorder but rather as a part of a group of symptoms that occur at the same time or in succession to each other. However, it is an important issue that needs to be documented and reported to determine the exact anxious disorder, or mental illness.

Medical professionals use the checklist for symptoms in order to figure out if the person's experience was actually panic attacks. The checklist lists symptoms that at least four of them must be present in the incident. Some of the symptoms mentioned include an increase in pulse rate, or heart palpitations. Also, there is a lot of sweating shaking or trembling feeling breathless or feeling shaky, chest pain or discomfort, anxiety, lightheadedness or dizziness, not being in the reality of the self, anxiety about being a liar and losing all control anxiety of dying and feeling numb (usually of extremes) and sensitivity to temperature.

The body's fight or flight mechanism activates whenever you are experiencing an anxiety attack. Nervous impulses released by the brain trigger the release of hormones, including adrenaline and epinephrine. These hormones cause the physical manifestations can be felt when experiencing panic attacks. Another factor that can be aggravating during an attack of panic is hyperventilation. This can make the symptoms worse , and could cause stress and anxiety.

It is usually triggered that triggers the initial panic attack. However, subsequent attacks could occur without warning or just for no reason. They can occur when you think you might have another attack. The symptoms you're experiencing cause you to feel more stressed. Although panic attacks usually gone in a matter of minutes however, you may experience several episodes of anxiety.

The tendency to suffer from anxiety attacks or panic disorders can be traced to genetics. A stressful and demanding life and experiencing traumas and difficulties throughout your life may cause you to be more prone to panic attacks.

What to Do When You Experience a Panic Attack

Contrary to the feeling of utter controllessness that you may experience when experiencing panic attacks it is actually you who are the most effective individual to stop an attack in it's source. Don't let the anxious and anxious thoughts take over your thoughts. While the panic attack may occur in a flash, you can just immediately clear out your thoughts and feelings that are causing the anxiety .

Being aware of your breathing is the first step to calm your mind and regaining control over your thoughts. Make sure you are prepared to practice deep breathing exercises you can begin when you feel the beginning of a panic attack. Concentrate on breathing slowly taking deep breaths and exhaling deeply. It is possible to count silently when you exhale and inhale. You can feel the air flowing into your body as it fills up your lung. Release the air slowly and feel all tension and worries being pulled out of your body. Repeat this process for a couple of minutes and you'll notice that the panic attack is gone.

Another method to combat anxiety attacks is to learn about your own body and identify the physical symptoms are evident when you're experiencing an attack. This will allow you to convince yourself that the symptoms you're experiencing is only temporary, that you're not really in danger and that there's no reason to be concerned.

If you are frequently experiencing anxiety attacks, it is possible that you be suffering from an anxiety disorder. In this case you must seek treatment. The most effective approach to treating anxiety disorders is to combine of cognitive behavior therapy and medication. Since the last few years it has been recognized as one of the most popular alternative treatments.

Chapter 11: What Is Anxiety?

Anxiety is a type of disorder that causes anxiety and stress, worry, anxiety, and fear within your body. It's the name used for certain disorders that affect the way a person feels and may cause physical signs. Anxiety that is mild can cause people feel uncomfortable, while an extreme anxiety could seriously impact the daily lifestyle of a person.

The United states of America, nearly 40 million Americans suffer by anxiety conditions. They are among the most prevalent kinds of mental illness across the nation. Yet, only around 37 percent of those affected by anxiety disorders receive the treatment they need.

Anxiety is a feeling that is characterised by a feeling of anxiety, worries and a rise in blood pressure. There's a vast distinction between anxiety that is normal and anxiety disorder that is so severe that it may require medical attention.

If a person encounters the threat of something or someone experiencing anxiety, it is normal, but it is also essential to live. From the beginning that predators used to to attack the victim, anxiety-related feelings were felt throughout the body, causing the victim suffer from anxiety disorders. An anxiety disorder may result in a heightened heart rate along with sweating that is more intense and very sensitive to the environment.

When someone is confronted with these anxiety disorders, a surge of adrenaline triggers a reaction to the actions. This adrenaline reaction is known as the "fight or flee" reaction. It causes a person to be prepared to confront or escape from dangers that are coming its way.

With time the anxiety disorders altered their course. They no longer fear of predators at work and money, family members health, as well as other issues that demand an individual's attention, without needing to engage in a fight or flight response.

Anxiety is a common type of disorder, and you may experience anxiety that is more severe and persistent in some instances. It can become overwhelming and difficult to control in some instances too. If it's extremely disturbing or irritating and causes an obstruction in daily activities, then it should be something that needs to be looked at.

Anxiety disorders can be serious medical conditions that are often as severe as diabetes and heart disease. There is a distinction between anxiety that is normal and disorder. While normal anxiety is normal and is common for people who experience it every day but anxiety disorders can be more serious and may require medical treatment and in some cases, hospitalization too.

Everyday anxiety:

Everyday stress includes worries about paying your bills, breaking up with your partner, losing an employment opportunity, and many other things in your life.

* finding yourself in awkward situations and being embarrassing in a crowd people

A lot of sweating prior to an exam or performance on stage or another crucial occasion

• Fearing of potentially dangerous object, creature, or scenario

* Sadness and anxiety are often associated by sleep problems following trauma

Anxiety disorder:

* A continuous worry that can cause stress and disruption throughout the day

* Avoiding social interactions or making new friends out of fear of being embarrassed, feeling left out, or being considered a failure

* A sudden panic attacks, and frequently anxiety disorders because of the worry of a panic attack

* A type of fear that is not rationally triggered by the object or animal

* terrifying nightmares, flashbacks to the past, memories of an old memory that could have changed your life in the last few months

Researchers have come to the conclusion that anxiety anxiety disorders are common in families with having a genetic basis like those of diabetes or allergies.

Anxiety disorders can result by a variety of risk factors, like genetics or brain chemistry, personality and life events that are significant.

Chapter 12: How To Prevent Depression And Anxiety Relapse

"Relapses "relapse" is when the symptoms of anxiety and depression are reappear after having overcome them. This is a fact, and at times, it's more severe. It is good to know that you have the ability to take steps to prevent the relapse from happening. Be aware that no one can assure that you'll never experience again unwell. However, the best part is that you're in a position to recognize the signs that indicate a problem and take action to address it. These tips can assist you in identifying the issue before symptoms develop into an actual problem. They can also help to reduce the impact of the symptoms on your daily life.

To avoid the possibility of relapse following your lengthy struggle with anxiety and depression Here are some good suggestions you can adhere to:

Part 1: Identifying and Being Aware Of the Early Warning Signs

This is the signal that suggests your health may be declining and again. This is one of usually the first warning signs that will appear before more serious symptoms begin to take a toll on your daily life. The reason you should categorize your distinct warning signs is to assist you in deciding to get it addressed in the earliest time possible.

Recognizing the warning signs early could make people feel anxious. In the end, no one would like to think about difficult or unpleasant circumstances.

In order to identify any warning indicators that appear in the first place, you must take a look back at the times when you struggled with anxiety and depression. Find out how it began and how it progressed in the course of your life, how you felt and what thoughts formed inside your head and what changes in your behavior took place. It can also be helpful to ask others around whether they have noticed any changes in you.

Part 2: Taking Action

After you've learned how to spot indications and signs that you should keep an eye on, it's now time to determine the best way to respond in the event that they occur. The following are the steps you must take to do:

Clear your mind. Begin by accepting. Whatever the cause is behind your depression or anxiety, you must keep in mind that it's not your responsibility. Perhaps you didn't have a positive childhood. Perhaps you're naturally sensitive. Maybe you've experienced something traumatizing. Even if you aren't at fault, it's important to recognize that it is your responsibility to correct the problem in order to make your life more enjoyable. Although anxiety and depression may be difficult to manage, you can attempt to overcome it. Instead of focusing on the negative idea, try thinking about the present. Let go of thoughts about the past that cause depression, and let go of the future that causes the future. Instead, focus on the present.

Develop your body. There was a time when you were trying to recover from anxiety and depression However, to avoid a return, you must repeat the process. Everyday life is filled with strains and pressures, which increases the allostatic burden and keeps the body free of negative emotions and moods. This effect can be further exacerbated by anxiety and increase the vulnerability of anxiety and depression. To reduce the stress make sure you get enough rest and exercise regularly be mindful of drinking too much or smoking, and also know how to manage your negative emotions to reduce anxiety. Keep this up until you feel better.

Change your anxiety and depression habits. Combating the issue is the opposite of avoiding. It's a simple fact. For a lot of people, the physical signs and negative emotions of anxiety and depression appear as if managing these issues is difficult to tackle. But, this method could be the most effective way to do to conquer a negative anxiety. Even if you don't think you're able to deal with the issues, you should plan an approach procedure where you develop steps that are to take a look at the things you normally avoid. Plan your approach as a series of actions to try that will result in an outcome that is positive.

Chapter 13: Coping With Socially Anxious Symptoms

If you're thinking "Hurry up and teach me how to get rid of my social anxiety already" and you've had enough of that dull theory from previous chapters, we'll get to that. This chapter will help you'll discover ways to manage anxiety. In this chapter, we will explore techniques for relaxation and shifting our focus as the first step to ease anxiety in a social context.

Relaxation

If you find yourself in a social gathering take a break and relax. Then, you will find occasions to be less stressful. What if you "just relax"? This could be the most unwise advice I've ever given. The purpose of this book is to show you how to enjoy social situations. Do not just to say "just relax". It's difficult for someone who is anxious to relax with the touch of a button. Unfortunately, you've probably been told this many times by those who do not suffer from social anxiety. I've seen this happen to me often. I'm sure the intentions of those who made this happen were good however, telling me to relax was absolutely useless. If I could be relaxed, I would not be suffering from social anxiety at all in the first instance.

Let's talk about the facts. Socializing in a relaxed way is extremely beneficial. It will reduce our social anxiety and help us become less focused on our own needs. When we feel nervous in social situations we don't feel relaxed. We feel stressed and anxious. It is evident from the signs you feel including heart rate racing quickly, muscle tension, rigid and stiff movement of your body, etc. As we have discussed previously in our chapter these signs can lead to a loop of stress, and you can are left feeling more stressed and anxious.

If we are relaxed, our stress and anxiety levels are much easier to manage. If we are relaxed it is evident that we can manage our social anxiety better. When we learn to relax in social settings it helps us manage our anxiety around social situations. Our anxiety is shown who's the boss!

The issue? Relaxing isn't an easy task. There aren't many who are able to completely unwind on the spot anytime they'd like. Particularly when they're anxious. However, it is possible. People who practice yoga, meditation and other forms of spirituality can unwind and appear at peace with their world. We can take a few techniques from them to ease our anxiety about social situations.

The Slow Breathing Technique

It is among the first things you'll discover when you visit the social phobia psychologist or sign up for an CBT program. The concept behind the Slow breathing technique is to intentionally reduce your breathing when you are in social situations, in order to dramatically reduce some physical manifestations associated with social anxiety.

If you're anxious in social situations the rate of your breathing tends to be quite quick. This may help to reinforce the fight or flight reaction, and trigger physical sensations.

There is a possibility the moment you talk your voice can be very rushed, and you might be exhausted. Similar to trying to speak at the conclusion of a running race. When someone would ask me "How did you find this place?" I would tend to answer "Uh..um.. alrigh- I mean uh.., I've comehereacoupletimesanduhyeahsoI'mus edtoit". Near the end of the my voice would become somewhat tense when I realized that I lost my voice. It was probably due to my fast breathing, which was exhausting me in a way that wasn't needed.

If we intentionally slow our breathing, the physical signs of anxiety decrease almost immediately. We do not feel as stressed when we are anxious and we aren't a socially anxious person before other people. The vicious cycle could get smashed. It will be apparent that you'll be more able to put your thoughts into your head and you will be less likely to experience panic attacks.

Here's the Slow Breathing method that you can attempt to do:

Breathe slowly and deeply through the nose for about 4 seconds. Be sure to breathe to the depth of your stomach.

Keep your breath in for 2 seconds.

Breathe slowly for four seconds.

Keep your breath for two seconds.

These numbers are just an example. There's no need to adhere to the 4-2-4-2 second rule with a strict adherence or else you'll never overcome anxiety about social situations. The idea is to intentionally and consciously make yourself breathe slower. Your subconscious might prompt you to breathe faster and it's your responsibility to calm it down and take charge. If you're comfortable doing something like 3-3-1 seconds, then try this instead. In general, 6-8 breathing cycles per minute is thought to be normal and relaxing. If you're getting more than 8 breath cycles per minute, then you're breathing too quickly. The average breathing rate is 12-18 cycles per minute. More than 20 breathing cycle per minute you're probably hyperventilating.

I would suggest you do this on your own. You can practice this in your home bedroom or anywhere you feel the most relaxed. It is recommended to learn this at home prior to when you do it in a stressful social setting. It is equally important to practice it regularly. at least twice a every day at a time for 10 minutes. Continue doing this until it becomes routine to you. Once you've established this habit, you may attempt it in a socially anxious setting.

Practice! Practice! Practice! You'll never be able to rest for a long time in the event that you did it for a day. It has to be an established habit within you. It is dependent on the person , but I would suggest giving it about one month before you start to see the outcomes. Then you will begin feeling a sense of relief whenever you're in a social context. Additionally, you will begin to feel as though you are in some way in ability to manage your anxieties. This is a great thing.

This is the homework assignment during this time. Test this for a week prior to when you start the next chapters and examine how you fare. If you are lucky you're doing this, it's working quite well. Take a couple of additional weeks, and perhaps attempt this in a social setting that you think is scary. It shouldn't be too difficult. It's not like going in front of someone and engage in conversations. I'm suggesting you do what you normally do, but now you intentionally slow your breathing whenever you feel uncomfortable.

Let Go!

Another method to relax and overcome your social anxiety. The idea behind this is to literally "let go" of all anxiety whenever you notice that it's there. Let's examine what this means:

Pay attention to the amount of muscle tension. Then determine if you feel tension, or if you're at ease.

Release all tension from your body and remind yourself to relax. Also, whenever you feel that there is tension in your body, let it go completely. You'll be like an uninteresting ragdoll body.

Perform this frequently all day long. Make sure to do it regularly and not just when you feel anxious.

There are a variety of ways to release tension in your body include:

Lowering your shoulders and hands and let them fall.

Then, you can place your head back on the headrest portion on the back of the chair.

Giving your legs space.

Sighing.

Breathing slowly (as we have mentioned).

Speak slowly to yourself to tell all over the universe "Relax".

Another exercise I observed to be extremely popular is when you purposely tension your body for a short period of time, then release and relax the body (on say, the number 3). You could, for instance, squeeze your fists as tightly as you can, and then instantly relax after you count 3.

As with similar to Slow Breathing method, you must also be able to practice regularly and practise! If you keep practicing the more likely it is that you'll be relaxed faster. It is recommended to first practice this at home before moving to social settings.

Don't expect to be relaxed if your do not consistently practice. It is possible to fail several times before you master these methods however the good thing is that you'll eventually begin being relaxed and break that vicious circle.

As a homework assignment I would suggest that you begin studying this technique. This means, you start by consciously clenching your fist after which you can begin "letting go" by releasing the fist. Do this for one week. Then , try doing this using your entire body. Tensify your entire body, and hold it as this. Let go, and slump down on your chair, like an uninterested dolly. If you do this repeatedly during the course of your day this can allow you to feel more at ease and calm when you are in social settings. Then, you can test this out in stressful social situations.

The primary goal of the Slow Breathing method and The Let Go technique, is that you discover how to be relaxed and pinpoint where the tension in your body is to let it go. This will allow you to release it and be much easier.

Other Ways To Feel Relaxed

You shouldn't be thinking about social anxieties or even your social daily. You must take some the time to be with yourself. Your best friend in life is actually you, If you consider it. You're always there to help you in the tough and the thin of occasions. It is important to respect yourself and indulge yourself to the max you can. The thought of social anxiety or methods to ease your social anxiety may be very draining and demotivating. In times of stress, we wish to be free of all of that and enjoy life.

There are a variety of ways to accomplish this and help to be more relaxed are:

You are thinking about the things that help you relax. Examples are walking by the sea, looking at the sun setting at the park in your neighborhood while playing music spending time with family or being excited about the latest trailer for your favorite actors ' new film.

Relax your posture when in social settings. Also you should be relaxed and not worry about. Tension doesn't look great, especially when we appear to be fixed to the ground, like statues.

Relax in a hot shower at the conclusion every day.

Movies watching.

The road is a blur.

Gardening.

Engaging in a sport or exercising.

And the list goes on. However, make sure you are at ease.

I find that being in a park with nature and fresh air helps to ease my anxiety and makes me feel less anxious. I also like watching a film at the close of the week. it gives me something to look forward to every week! I also like watching YouTube videos and listening to music. If you are doing things that make you feel relaxed then you'll be more relaxed and not fret about anxiety as much. Being involved in the activities you enjoy can increase your confidence.

Shift Attention Away

When you're in a social setting that you consider to be uncomfortable You may be thinking about the physical symptoms or what other people might consider about your appearance. When you think about what others may think of your behavior, you are likely to be self-conscious and fear the worst about their reactions. If their reactions are more severe as you had feared and you are not prepared, it can cause you to lose your mind. When you keep looking for reactions from others it can make you feel uneasy and unsure of who you are and would be unable to deal with this situation within a planned way. If you recall the lessons learned, considering the reaction of others can create an unending cycle that keeps our anxiety about social situations running.

What if we explore ways to break this cycleand divert ourselves from thoughts that aren't our own. This makes sense in the theory, doesn't it? Instead of thinking constantly negatively about things (like "What if I stuff up?", "What if they think I'm weird") We make ourselves feel better by thinking about random things (like "Oh that chair is blue, never saw a blue chair before", or "Am I the shortest person here?"). ?"). When you think like this your mind doesn't know think of what to make out from your thoughts and won't make you feel nervous. Instead, your anxiety will reduce.

It's possible that this is easier to say than done. It's true. You may consciously think about random thoughts however in your head, you can't help but hear the voice that says "What if...what if...what do you think? ...". Similar to techniques like Slow Breathing or Let Go techniques, it's just a matter of the practice. After you've learned to shift your focus a lot and you'll find it easy to handle your anxiety. Imagine a child who is very playful. I can picture his mother screaming and shouting at him to not or, I'm not sure, hit a button or anything. The mind may be elsewhere, and in the next second, he's attempting to hit that button once more. While a highly sensitive person may be afraid to press the button due to that panicked reaction. One reason to this is that the child, possibly because of his age, is a bit distracted and was so distracted by other things. He never was able to resist doing again. The person who is sensitive may be thinking about the button and worry about the possibility of hitting it. Although I don't believe that having a shorter attention span as an issue but I wanted to illustrate how thoughts that are distracted can affect how we feel.

Let's take a look at ways to stay occupied in social settings without looking rude:

Be aware of what's happening in the scene. You can count the chairs that are within the space, figure out who's age as well as the height you're relative to the rest of the group or count how many girls and boys are in the room, and other things like that. This will force you to concentrate on the outside rather than the things you're experiencing within yourself.

Get busy doing something. If you have something you want to do then you'll be focused on the task, not your own needs.

Ask questions. If you ask questions, you draw focus away from you and the person talking. You shouldn't continue asking them questions, as they don't want to appear like they're being questioned by the police.

Of course, there's an important distinction between safety and distraction. If you are trying to distract yourself by playing on your phone even though you're distracting your mind, you are still engaging in a safety practice that can cause anxiety.

Try using distraction in times of stress or in a social setting. Be sure to not be distracted by your thoughts or you could be perceived as unprofessional and unprofessional.

Summary

In this chapter, we discussed ways to deal with social anxiety. We looked at relaxation methods. Two methods we examined included those that involve the

Slow Breathing technique where we deliberately slow the pace of our breathing to lessen physical symptoms as well as The Let Go technique where we get stiff and tense in your body, and then let go. We also examined shifting your focus away from our anxiety-provoking thoughts to end the cycle known as social Anxiety. The next section will provide a detailed method of getting over social anxiety.

Chapter 14: About Antidepressants

The use of medications can combat depression and anxiety. For instance, antidepressants can stabilize and normalize brain's neurotransmitters, including serotonin, norepinephrine and dopamine. These neurotransmitters are crucial because they control mood.

Selective serotonin-reuptake inhibitors, also known as SSRIs are the most sought-after forms of antidepressants. They comprise Zoloft, Prozac, and Celexa.

Norepinephrine Reuptake inhibitors, also known as SNRIa, are like SSRIs. They comprise Cymbalta along with Effexor. These antidepressants are less likely to cause adverse effects compared to antidepressants of the past such as tricyclics or monoamine oxidase inhibitors, or MAOIs.

MAOIs are great for those who suffer from adverse side effects from taking SNRIs and SSRIs. They are, however, MAOIs should be taken with caution as they could cause significant interactions with specific drugs and food items. Pickles, wine, and cheeses include large amounts of tyramine which could interact with MAOIs that's the reason why they should be avoided.

There are decongestants too that contain the chemical tyramine. They should therefore be avoided too. Note that when tyramine is in contact with MAOI and blood pressure, an increase and strokes may occur. Patients taking MAOIs must also receive an inventory of foods or substances should be avoided for the sake of avoiding uncomfortable negative side negative effects.

If you're using antidepressants, there may be no noticeable changes until after several weeks of using. It is important to be patient with your outcomes and don't stop the use of these medications. Also, ensure that you are taking the correct dosage. It is essential to not do more or less than the prescribed dose by your physician. with.

Don't cut off your medication even if you feel better. You should stop taking the medication when your physician has instructed you to. Antidepressants are effective in improving the condition of your body and can also stop your from suffering from a repeat or repeating. If you believe that you must quit taking these drugs and consult with your physician.

If you are taking antidepressants you must be monitored to ensure that you do not suffer from withdrawal symptoms. The body is not able to easily adjust to changes, which is why it is necessary to take your patience. While antidepressants aren't typically addictive, you could suffer from unpleasant side effects if they stop your treatment abruptly.

If you are concerned that your antidepressants don't work You should inform your doctor. Ask him to recommend a different medication. According to studies, treatments can be more effective if patients change from a drug which isn't working to a different one.

The side effects of antidepressants are typically short-term and minor. The long-term effects of antidepressants are uncommon. However, you should not be reluctant to speak to your physician if you experience any strange reactions or side effects. Medical supervision is required when you have extreme adverse reactions.

What are the most common side effects patients can experience when taking SSRIs or SNRIs? The headache and nausea is the most common side effect experienced by patients who first began using these medicines. Fortunately, these symptoms disappear over time. It is common for people to experience agitation as well.

Patients might be afflicted with insomnia or have difficulty sleeping. If you're taking these medicines and have trouble sleeping after a few weeks of use You can request your physician to lower the dosage. For males Erectile dysfunction can also occur.

On the other hand those who take tricyclic antidepressants usually have dry mouth, constipation low libido, blurred vision and daytime sleepiness. Some men may also experience Erectile dysfunction that is delayed or delayed. People with larger prostates might struggle to empty their bladders.

Additionally, suicidal tendencies may develop. This is particularly the case for adolescents and children who take antidepressants. Certain antidepressants may trigger suicidal thoughts and behavior. Therefore, a close monitoring is essential during the initial couple of weeks after treatment.

The warning signs must also be taken note of by health care specialists. They can be a sign of suicidal thoughts and behavior changes, insomnia or social withdrawal, as well as an agitation. However, despite these negative effects, medical professionals continue to advise antidepressants because of their effectiveness in managing depression and anxiety.

Chapter 15: Treatments For Social Anxiety Disorder

The first step to treat depression and anxiety disorders is to recognize that you are suffering from a disorder. It is then time getting assistance. Recognizing and accepting that something isn't right isn't easy. Early detection and treatment are vital.

There are medicines, such as antidepressants, which could be beneficial. But, there are effective ways you can manage and ultimately beat SAD which don't require prescription drugs.

Challenge Your Negative Thoughts

The majority of the time negative thoughts can trigger symptoms of anxiety and fear. If you suffer from SAD you may be overwhelmed by the negative thoughts and beliefs:

* "They might laugh at me."

*"I may not be adequate."

*"They may think I'm dumb."

*"I do not know the right words to use."

* "I'm afraid my voice will shake and everyone will know how nervous I am."

The most effective way to conquer those negative beliefs is to try to overcome these thoughts. Therapy sessions or perform it yourself. For example, if you are worried about being laughed at while you speak, substitute the negative thoughts with encouraging phrases like "I am good and well-prepared and they are going to love me." Then, challenge your negativity by asking: "How sure are you to be sure they'll laugh? Give three specific examples" Control negative thoughts and eliminate them.

Practice Breath Control

If you're stressed you may feel a heavy breathing that could cause an increase in the heart rate and muscle tension, as well as dizziness , and a sense of being suffocated. Learn breathing exercises that ease anxious symptoms. You can do relaxation activities you can try. Yoga is also a great exercise that will aid in learning to breathe effectively when you're stressed and anxiety. It is also possible to explore meditation and techniques for relaxation of muscles.

If you notice difficulty breathing, inhale slowly and exhale repeatedly until your breathing is back to normal.

Learn to Face Your Fears

Doctors advise their patients to face their fears if they wish to conquer these fears. If you continue to avoid your fears, you'll not be able to get beyond them. Although avoiding the issues you are facing can help you feel better, it's an ineffective solution for the short-term. Refraining from problems can cause more discomfort in any social context. It's not a way to learn anything. Be aware that the longer you are unable to confront fear, the more terrifying they will become.

If you try to avoid the fear, then you allow your fears rule your. When confronting your fears be aware that you don't need to make yourself face your most feared fears right away. Slow down and be patient. It takes time and consistent practicing. Start small and take it one step at an time.

Begin Building Better Relationships

One of the most effective ways to get over social anxiety is to venture out and start interacting with people. It is possible to start by attending a class on social skills taught at the community adult educational center or the community college. Participate in your church's activities or any other event within your community that will require interaction with others.

Make Changes in Your Lifestyle

Making a few adjustments to how you live could aid the treatment process overall. Eliminating anxiety and stress by reducing your intake of caffeine. Consume alcohol in moderation. Some people drink alcohol as It calms the nerves. However, alcohol can trigger panic attacks as well. You should consider quitting smoking as Nicotine is an stimulant and can cause anxiety to rise. You must ensure that you have enough sleep. Lack of sleep makes people more susceptible to anxiety and panic attacks.

Get Professional Help

If you find these self-help techniques to be ineffective then it is recommended to seek out a professional. There are many ways to help overcome your social anxiety. A highly effective methods can be cognitive behavioral therapy. This therapy focuses on observing how your thoughts influence your reactions to certain situations. It helps you alter your thinking about social situations that can trigger anxiety attacks. It can also help to manage physical symptoms by teaching relaxation methods. It can help you learn to manage social situations with a plan, so you don't become overwhelmed by too many changes all at once.

Medications

The use of medication can help ease the effects, yet they do not completely eliminate social anxiety. They are most effective if they are used in conjunction with therapy at the same at the same time.

Types of Medication That May Help With Social Anxiety

*Antidepressants can be helpful particularly when symptoms become chronic. There are a variety of medications which are recognized from The US Food and Drug Administration that doctors prescribe.

*Beta blockers are prescribed as a way to ease of symptoms of performance anxiety. They block the flow of adrenaline that is elevated during an anxiety attack. Beta blockers are able to address physical signs like a fast heartbeat, shaking, and sweating.

*Benzodiazephines are drugs that are quick-acting and act as sedatives. But, these medications are also addictive. This is why they are prescribed after all other medications not alleviate anxieties about social situations do not work.

Chapter 16: Treating Social Anxiety

Social anxiety is a major factor in the lives of 19.2 million people each year. Sadly, this number is currently growing and is not expected to decline in the near future.

Social phobia usually develops at an early age and, if it is not addressed, could quickly turn into a complete mental disorder when teenagers are approaching.

It is the second most frequent anxiety disorder and is also the third most prevalent mental disorder, behind alcoholism and depression. may be combined with social anxiety and create an unfavorable combination.

Social anxiety is reported twice as often than in men, according to research conducted by Cambridge University. University of Cambridge.

The above facts are alarming and the fact that social anxiety when left untreated could cause panic attacks, extreme depression and, in certain cases, suicide. is enough to make you want to get to the root of it once all and come up with an answer.

There are a variety of alternatives to address your anxiety about social situations, such as the use of professional therapy, medications to reduce anxiety or seeking out professional assistance to manage their disorder.

If you are working with psychiatrists or psychologists you are receiving treatment from an expert who is trained to diagnose and treat mental disorders.

There are two primary kinds of treatment for social anxiety that your therapist can use:

Cognitive Behavior Therapy (CBT) CBT CBT involves training the brain to view your thoughts and feelings regarding social situations in a different way. It is extensively used by therapists across the world to assist patients in making permanent changes in the way they handle social interactions with other people.

Medication - Medicines such as beta-blockers and antidepressants, as well as anti-anxiety medications like Paxil are commonly utilized by people suffering from shyness and social anxiety. A lot of people have noticed positive improvements because of the use of these medicines, while many complain about the negative consequences that can result from their usage.

There is another type therapy for people suffering from social anxiety called NLP also known as neuro-linguistic programing. It has been demonstrated to deliver impressive results but isn't as well-known for cognitive therapy. This will not be discussed by this guide.

It is crucial to consult a physician before you take medication, and seek out therapy with a licensed doctor. They are better equipped to prescribe the right dosage of the medication and assist you in overcoming your anxiety.

Managing Your Symptoms

The treatment process can be a long time before becoming efficient, and in some cases it's an ongoing process. Based on how serious your symptoms are, it could take longer . Therapy might have to be an everyday procedure. A lot of patients are unable to afford private treatment or medication. There are a variety of self-help techniques available to those clients as therapy is expensive. Do not give up and keep to it, sooner or later, you'll see results.

Chapter 17: Take Charge Of Your Message

Are you aware of The Law of Attraction? It is one of the Universal concepts that deal with the idea that, in the world of life, "like attracts like". The sayings "birds of a feather flock together" and "the apple doesn't fall far from the tree" all affirm this notion.

The LOA says that everything in the universe is energy. All of us operate on particular frequencies. The things and people we are currently surrounded by are an example of our current mental state. "Misery loves company"- this is another one that's good.

Have you seen someone always down? They were the typical "glass half empty thinker". What did they affect you? Uncomfortable? Frustrated? This is because your personality wasn't in sync with yours.

Be The CEO

You , as the owner of your brand are in the position to determine who you draw and how they perceive your message. Beginning with your visualization and your visualization, you'll begin to feel excited about your presentation. This enthusiasm will spread into your speech and what you say as well as your nonverbal communication. The final lessons should make you aware of things such as tone, speed and your body language. Enhancing your self-confidence will have helped you overcome your mistakes to this point. Make sure that your presentation is on standards.

The Introduction: The first impressions you make last. Research shows that the first two minutes of your presentation are the only time you need to get the attention of your audience and maintain it. What can you do to achieve this? Beginning with your presentation, you language are supposed to be compelling and instructive. Tell them what you'll be offering them , without saying, "Today we're going to talk about self-confidence." Be imaginative!

Begin by telling a short tale. A situation that has occurred to you or someone else. Retell a story of things you've conquered or things you're fighting with. The stories you tell will make you feel emotional, and emotions can be a source of understanding. From the top executive to the entry-level worker Everybody's been hurt, everyone's felt some joyEstablish a shared base.

Shock is a great alternative. The Bill Gate presentation that was among his most infamous T.E.D. presentation was about Malaria. The speaker began the presentation by releasing mosquitoes to the audience. Do you think of the reaction? The reaction was shocking. It's memorable. It was pertinent. It stirred emotions.

Slides and Charts - A popular choice to many speakers, but as technology advances however, the use of the traditional slide is disapproved of. If you have to use slides be sure to not overload them with unnecessary information. Make sure to highlight the most important points and expand on them your own. Your audience won't need to be reading paragraphs of information. Based on their understanding and pace of the presentation excessive text can create space for facts to get lost in the process of translation. This shouldn't occur. If you're forced to make use of media, videos are far more efficient. You can still incorporate actual facts while also grabbing the attention of your audience.

Humor - What was once an option now is seen as a necessity. Inspire your audience to laugh and you'll have them paying attention. This is a tricky chance to make in particular if you're not especially humorous. Don't make jokes about stand-up comedy. Instead, you should try to write an entertaining story. It could be about your own life or about someone you've met. If it's something you and your colleagues might laugh about during work (and it's pertinent to your topic) Don't be shyand share the joke with your group.

Timing is Everything - Long past are the times when you were obliged to endure painful 2-hour-long presentations. According to T.E.D. experts, the statistics indicate that you should aim for 18 minutes as the ideal time frame. What can I do to talk about a year's worth of research in only 18 minutes? The process of reduction is the most appealing aspect of this process. In only 18 seconds, our brain used all of its capability. Retention and processing of new information is not easy. Do you remember those long hours in school? You'd be exhausted when you got home as if you'd constructed an entire house from scratch for seven hours. The brain is extremely active. Take note of it's capabilities. You'd rather spend an hour giving the speech of the decade, rather than taking up the time of all people.

If you are going to exceed the suggested 18-minute time limit, make sure you provide your audience with mental breaks. Take breaks to share stories, or show videos, or ask questions. Give your brain time to relax before proceeding to the next section.

Keep your PromiseWhat you said in your introduction must be fully covered when you're done speaking. Do not tell your audience that you'll show them how you can make more money by selling insurance, and then forget to refer to insurance once more. Make sure you are clear on your goals and then present. If your audience leaves with questions, the focus must be focused on what's to come next. They shouldn't ever feel that they didn't get what were expecting.

Chapter 18: Anxiety Self-Help

Self-help anxiety tip 1

Set up a worry-free period

The people who suffer from anxiety depression are unable to remain productive and to concentrate on their personal and social lives. They often feel anxious and anxious about events that may happen or have already happened. The mind is busy and they are unable to complete their tasks in a timely manner. The best self-help for anxiety for these people is to create the condition of worry.

How can you create a worrying period

The process of creating a worry-free period is an easy task that you can accomplish by deciding on a particular moment in the day and contemplating all the issues you have during that period. It should not last more than twenty or thirty minutes. This should be enough time to reflect on your issues and consider the solutions. The time of worry should remain the same throughout the day. It is not recommended to prolong your worry period prior to going to bed because you'll be thinking about your problems and may have difficulty sleeping.

Delay your worries

If at any time you have a worry-inducing thought in your thoughts, do not be aware of it. It is best to put it off for a later time. If you've established a specific your time frame for becoming anxious and undergoing anxiety stress it is best not to spend your entire day worry.

If you begin managing your anxiety by contemplating them at a certain date and time, you'll also be able to master control your anxiety. When you can see that you can postpone your worries according to your wishes, then you'll begin to gain control over these worries.

Self-help for anxiety - Tip 2

Examining if the issue can be resolved

According to research, those who are more anxious tend to become stressed and feeling less anxious when they are worried. However, it is crucial to understand that worrying won't solve any problem. There is a distinct distinction between worrying and problem solving. Rethinking the issue over and again is not going to resolve it.

The difference in worrying and solution

The people who are suffering from anxiety stress fail to realize that putting stress on themselves will not help them. Problem solving is a distinct ability. It is the process of contemplating a particular issue and determining the root of the issue and determining its effect, developing a strategy to address the issue. In the process of worrying, the individual is unable to find a solution to the issue. For those who are worried, they should search for anxiety self-help

The process of identifying solvable and nonsolvable issues

If you have something that is bothering you, it is best to take the time to reflect on the issue. There are two kinds of issues that people could be confronted with:

Solvable and insolvable

The problem that can be solved is the one you're currently facing at this moment.

Unsolvable problem is one that you've assumedproblems that begin by asking "what if". Unsolvable issues are forever-lasting and originate from the mind by your own imagination.

If you're in search of an anxiety relief, you must first establish whether your issue is real or are you making assumptions about it. If the problem is solvable, it has a solution. It is essential to tackle the issue and concentrate on the root of the issue and create plans. Start your plan as soon as possible in order to fix the issue. If, for instance, you are concerned of passing an exam, then you must be prepared for it. If you're worried about your husband not being there at some point in the future, or you developing cancer at some point in life, then this is something you are not able to control and is considered to be an impossible to solve.

Self-help with anxiety to solve unsolvable issues

If you're facing an issue that doesn't really exist, but is an outcome of your self-assumed thinking, then you're a suffering from depression and anxiety. Look for ways to help yourself to deal with the issue that is unsolvable.

If you allow the fear to over you, you'll never get rid of it. It will be a constant in your mind throughout your life. If you're worried about something that doesn't exist, and you believe that it will occur in the near future, you're not right. The only way to break out of the cycle of anxiety is to let go of your fears and letting them flow as they naturally do. Be aware that emotions can trigger negative feelings and even disturb your thoughts. To break from stress and anxiety, you must have an effective control of your feelings. Even if you are constantly worried about an issue that you cannot solve for a long time and devote the majority of your time to it there is no solution.

Anxiety self-help tips 3

Accept the possibility of uncertainty

People who are suffering from depression or anxiety are more likely to be concerned about things that aren't evident. They need to be sure that everything is in order. Even if they have thought of everything, they'll be contemplating it until the time comes. They need to know ahead of time what is the result of an action. They don't have a 99 percent or 98 percent. They require a one-cent assurance of all things prior to the event. They do not acknowledge that uncertainty is an integral aspect of life. However hard we try, we will never be 100% certain about any thing. Human life itself is uncertain , and no one knows how long he'll live to live another day.

Be prepared for the uncertainty

If you're seeking anxiety relief, then be able to manage anxiety. Accept the fact that it is a part of life. You should ask yourself these questions whenever you aren't able to get the perfect answer to an issue.

What is the reason I am concerned about something?

What is my primary issue?

Can an individual can be absolutely certain of?

What is the chance of a specific problem based on laws of average?

What if I thought about a specific negative event prevent it from happening?

Do I have a chance to get a warranty without worrying?

Does my worry do any positive things for my life?

Many people are observed to be concerned about the negative events that could occur in the near future. People forget that being worried about things that have not yet happened is not letting them enjoy the present moment in peace. They'll miss the wonderful times that life provides when they think about the negative things that could take place in the near future.

Self-help for anxiety - 4

Consider how other people impact your life

The individual has the full right to lead his own life, without worrying about others or their actions. In the family structure and in places where others have significant influence on one's life, many people are suffering from depression and anxiety. If, for instance, you live in a region with a rigid social structures and the people don't have enough freedom, the decisions you make in your life are influenced by what other people think of their opinions. If you wish to pursue the path of a particular profession or get married to an individual who is not part of your religion or social standing, you may not be able to achieve it. Someone who is suffering from anxiety will always be worried about what people around him are thinking about and how his actions and behavior influence those surrounding them. It is essential to understand the self-help advice for anxiety to work , you should be able to remove

162

yourself from social pressures and pressure from peers.

Follow your heart

The key to a fulfilling life is to follow the way you feel. If you spend too much time thinking about what other people think and think, you'll get stuck and never be able to progress with your goals. You should ask yourself these questions before you decide making an important decision.

Do I really need this?

Who will profit from my choice?

What will my decision have an impact on another person?

Does my specific act have an effect on others? If so, what happens?

Who is responsible for the choices I make?

Did any of my actions had an impact on someone else before? If not, how does it impact someone today?

Am I being realistic?

Do my concerns have a rational basis?

Does my worry alter something?

The people around you will share their views and some may be able to tell you how untrue you are, but in reality no one will be responsible for actions you make and the decisions you make and the decisions you make. People chat for a few minutes before returning to their lives. It's been so busy that there is no the time to contemplate what other people are doing. Everyone is focused on their own lives and tackling their own personal issues. If you're facing an issue, you are the only person to solve the problem. People are fond of talking about others , but no one will solve your problem.

Chapter 19: Controlling Anxiety Attacks

Are you constantly feeling anxious , without a reason? Do you feel anxious and anxious about certain events or people, places, or even things? There are several indicators that suggest you are suffering from an anxiety attack.

Also called panic attack, suffering from an anxiety attack can cause stress and can result in future issues in the event that they are not properly addressed. There are many efficient ways to ease anxiety before it becomes worse. Understanding the right techniques for managing anxiety will help you conquer anxiety.

The majority times, an anxiety attack isn't due to actual threats, rather by the mental state of the individual. Although it is common to feel anxious about an upcoming date examination or job interview, it's uncommon for a person to be overly anxious enough to lose the ability to function as a normal human being.

So, how can you minimize the possibility of being very in the grip of anxiety? There are many methods to achieve this.

In the first place, you need to recognize that seeking out professional help isn't a bad option. Many people avoid this possibility, believing that only people who have already"lost it" have to see a psychologist, but this isn't the case.

A trained professional therapist will offer practical solutions or, if required may even suggest treatments or medication. Your anxiety disorder could get to an extent where your the home remedies and other methods might not be effective anymore.

If you consult with an expert, you will be diagnosed correctly. The cause of your issue can be identified and addressed.

In the majority of cases doctors will advise that you adopt a healthy and balanced lifestyle. It's a fact that the majority of people who suffer from panic attacks don't get enough sleep. Relaxing your body is a great method to reduce anxiety and stress. This can help you feel more energized and excited as you try to tackle certain issues which you must deal with. Additionally exercising regularly is an effective way to reenergize your body as well as your mind. A lot of experts recommend this as an effective method to reduce anxiety attacks.

You can also consider relaxing techniques such as doing yoga or meditation. Like exercise, it will be beneficial to your body and mind. Research has proven that people who do yoga or meditate are less prone to suffering anxiety attacks than people who don't.

Furthermore, avoiding drinking alcohol is essential to get rid of anxiety and feelings of panic. Although many would like you to believe that alcohol consumption is antidepressants, they are contrary and you must be aware. Be especially cautious to avoid drinking alcohol during or following an anxiety attack since it can cause harm.

Diet is a major factor. Making sure you don't skip meals and adhering to a balanced diet will be beneficial to you. In particular, consider eating food high in magnesium and potassium. You'll be healthierand your risk of suffering from anxiety attacks will be significantly reduced.

Additionally, it is helpful to have a trusted friend who is willing to listen and provide helpful suggestions whenever you face problems. It is definitely helpful for you to possess an"emotional outlet" in the sense of having an outlet and having a partner (or colleague from the family) who you feel comfortable to speak to can have an impact on your efforts to ease anxiety.

Do not be afraid to seek advice from a physician If you believe you're not succeeding in your quest to conquer anxiety. There's no reason not to consult an expert psychologist. Psychologists are always willing to help and help you overcome anxiety.

Possible Treatments and Therapies

To get rid of the issue it is necessary to start making lifestyle changes that are healthy. Exercise can be a big aid, particularly when you exercise frequently. Meditation, yoga, stretching as well as massages are other treatments can be used to reduce the likelihood to suffer from anxiety-related attacks.

Consuming healthy foods can be an element. In particular, it is important to seek out foods which are high in potassium and magnesium. The best sources are sun-dried tomato, potatoes, cantaloupes, seaweeds cereals, nuts, raisins seafood, meat, and fish as well as other items.

Naturally, it's essential to stop smoking cigarettes, using recreational drugs, as well as drinking alcohol or coffee. These harmful substances can cause anxiety and stress, and it's better to stay clear of these substances.

A good night's rest is essential in being able to overcome anxiety. You'll feel less cranky If you sleep enough at night, therefore, make it a point to get at least between seven and nine hours sleep every day.

If you are determined to overcome anxiety You must develop a positive attitude about yourself. Being more confident and feeling confident about yourself can boost your self-esteem. This will help reduce the stress you feel. For this, think about using a notebook to write down what you admire about yourself. Do a self-evaluation of your personality, abilities and abilities. If you do this regularly you will reap enormous benefits.

A consultation with a professional is only recommended when you are experiencing extreme anxiety attacks. Psychologists can assist you in dealing problems and will recommend specific solutions, too. Treatments or medications will be recommended to ensure that you're able to deal with the issue. Most of the time it is necessary to see your doctor more than one time.

For more information on the causes of anxiety and what options for solving it are, reading books and looking through different websites is a good option. With these resources you will gain more knowledge and get useful tips from experts.

Chapter 20: Understanding Anxiety And Anxiety Disorders

Anxiety is the body's normal response to situations that could be life-threatening and should not be thought of as the source of your present problems. It's perfectly normal to be anxious when you're facing an extremely important event like meeting for the first time, performance in front of a large crowd, an interview or test. The anxious mechanism when functioning, can actually be very beneficial, as it allows the mind to switch its attention to the important occasion that is ahead of you. It makes your mind be more attentive, focused and perhaps even motivated and inspired.

But, too much of anything is harmful And as you are aware, anxiety isn't exempt from this.

Sometimes, we are more focused on our anxiety than we're focused on the thing that has caused anxiety in the beginning. Most of the time, we don't have the ability to pinpoint the cause that has caused our anxiety. This is where things get a little off track.

The standard definition for anxious disorders is to experience a overwhelming feeling of pressure and anxiety. It's above the normal anxiety level and doesn't fulfill its purpose that is to keep your mind focused and alert on important events or activities. In reality, excessive anxiety causes it to be difficult to be logical and focused on the most important issues.

Major classifications of anxiety disorders.

In the first place, it's essential to recognize that in our day and time anxiety disorders are fairly widespread. Studies show that they are the most frequent type of mental disease within the United States. It's so widespread, that many sufferers aren't aware about the possibility that they're suffering from anxiety disorders. The most common definition of anxious disorder refers to the inexplicably strong feeling of being scared or pushed, as well as anxious. There are a variety of types of anxiety disorders. The main classifications of anxiety disorders are obsessive-compulsive disorder(OCD), social anxiety disorder and post-traumatic stress disorder. panic disorder, or panic attacks and the phobias.

* Obsessive-compulsive disorder

Obsessive-compulsive disorder , also known as OCD is defined as anxiety-related disorder characterised by uncontrollable behaviors or thoughts. According to its name OCD is a disorder that afflicts its sufferer with continuous anxiety, which causes them to be obsessed with the specific action they are compelled to perform. The person suffering from OCD is terrified of the potential harm that could happen when the action of compulsive is not performed. A common symptom of obsessive compulsive disorder, such as is the constant and uncontrollable desire to wash your hands.

* Social anxiety disorders

People who suffer from a Social anxiety disorder constantly scared of being judged or criticized by others. They worry about being embarrassed in public. On the extreme, people who suffer from social anxiety disorder complete withdrawal from social interactions. The most well-known example of a disorder known as social anxiety is stage fright, also known as performance anxiety. Studies show that this fear can lead to the sky financial ruin, illness and even death.

* Post-traumatic Stress Disorder

Everyone is likely to experience an immense amount of stress following being exposed to a scary or life-threatening troubling or depressing event. Physical assault, sexual abuse or extreme violence or the loss of an individual's loved ones can cause tremendous pain and cause damage to the mental well-being of a person. In the majority of instances of post-traumatic stress, it is best to heal yourself and no treatment is required for those who have suffered from the trauma will heal all on his own. But, for some people the condition can become worse over time, and those who suffer from it are considered to be sufferers of the post-traumatic stress disorder or PTSD. The sufferers of PTSD can develop a heightened fear of any an entity that, whether conscious or not, recalls the traumatizing event they have experienced during the previous time.

* Panic disorder/Panic attacks

The human body's normal reaction to tension or stress. However, anyone suffering from an anxiety disorder is susceptible to an attack which causes extreme anxiety and anxiety. The level of anxiety and anxiety experienced by people suffering from an anxiety disorder isn't always in line with the circumstance; it likely isn't an actual threat. Someone who is experiencing panic attacks may manifest physical symptoms like nausea, physical pain and dizziness, or even excessive sweating.

* Phobias

Phobias may be the most diverse mental condition in medical history. They are described as having an unfounded and extreme fear of a particular thing, event or physical action. Phobias can be triggered by things that are the least harmful like cotton balls, buttons, or peaches. However, in most cases, they are more reasonable and easier to explain, including fears of spiders (Arachnophobia) and anxiety about flying (Aerophobia) and anxiety about being locked in and having no escape (Claustrophobia) and fear of high places (Acrophobia) and many others.

Physical and mental signs of anxiety disorders

* Irritability

* Restlessness

Always look for any warning signs

* Reduced attention span

* Being assertive and tense.

* Negative thinking that is uncontrollable

* Excessive sweating

* Insomnia

* Fatigue

* A loss of appetite

* Tension in the muscles

* Physical discomfort

* Breathing shortness

* Heart racing

Conclusion

In this stage you'll be able to channel your mindfulness whenever the situation requires it. The book's discussion has focused on ways you can improve your mindfulness to be able to use it effectively, in your everyday life.

As this book comes to an end This is a brief checklist to use in moments of stress. If you feel you're losing focus and are getting lost in the moment take these steps:

Step 1: Stop. In order to be able to channel the state of mind, you must take a moment to stop and then stop for a few seconds. Whatever you're doing or the condition you're in right now and you must be able to take a moment of rest. Sit down.

Step 2: Look. To fully be at the moment you must be aware of all that's happening around you. You can assume the role of witness. Remove yourself from the scene and look around.

Step 3: Assess. It's normal to feel a certain way about what's happening. Let yourself pass judgment however, let it go. Don't dwell on your decisions, but take an outline of your observations.

These three steps are essential in directing your mind to mindfulness. As you try to do this the mind naturally will wander and that's okay. The key to success in mindfulness is the ability to come back (again and repeatedly) in the current. It is necessary to repeat these three steps in order to be in a position to return to the present moment.

www.ingramcontent.com/pod-product-compliance
Lightning Source LLC
Chambersburg PA
CBHW060326030426
42336CB00011B/1216